Babyphobia

Dr. Tzachi Topelberg

⟨?⟩

Copyright © 2015
By Dr. Tzachi Topelberg
All rights reserved
ISBN: 1530292239
ISBN-13: 978-1530292233

TO MY PARENTS

I would like to thank the world that has presented me with so many obstacles and barriers in life. I had to choose: give up or prevail... and I prevailed.

I would like to thank all the people I met throughout my life, who encouraged me to be what I am today.

To my daughters, Adi and Shani, who grew up to be beautiful, talented women, who during the years, reflected my strength and my weaknesses back to me.

I wish to thank my late father and mother, who did their best to give me the tools for life, like any parents. I rebelled sometimes; however, in retrospect, I feel lucky I had my parents.

Babyphobia

Contents

Babyphobia

LET'S TALK ABOUT YOUR FUTURE BABY

Yes, you all have the right to become a mother, and do not let anyone tell you different.

Let me tell you a story that happened twenty-one years ago: I had a female friend; tests showed that her Fallopian tubes were blocked. The doctors, all of them top gynecologists, told her to give up on her dream; that if she wanted a child, she should adopt one, because medical knowledge at that time gave her a zero percent chance of her conceiving. Just a few days ago, her son celebrated his twentieth birthday. She conceived naturally, had very stable pregnancy and the baby was born healthy. When she asked the doctors, "How come?" they said, "We don't know."

This was not a miracle. Our minds are much stronger than we know, for better or for worse.

You will hear the same answer from your doctor after the failure of a round of IVF treatment. The statistics show a success rate in IVF procedures of just 14-35%. Why? The doctor inserts a fertile embryo to a woman's womb, but the healthy body rejects the embryo.

Do not let anyone give you any excuse why you do not conceive. Pregnancy can be the essence of a woman's existence. A baby can bring a pinnacle of happiness that no drug can match. For the last twelve years, I have helped many women to conceive. How? During my years of practice, I developed a method of treatment I call Rebound Psychotherapy. My aim is to quickly and efficiently help people suffering from anxieties, including fear of flying, agoraphobia, OCD, ADD, ADHD, and many others. I soon found out that many healthy women who came over to me for therapy conceived naturally during the therapy process. Initially, perhaps, they came for treatment for other anxieties, while in parallel they were planning to conceive or to undergo IVF. Soon enough, I realized that my Rebound Psychotherapy system can touch the places in the patient's mind that can prevent the body from conceiving. My findings showed that many healthy women do not conceive due to a mental barrier stopping the woman's reproductive system from working properly.

I would like to emphasize that when I refer to a "healthy woman," I mean a woman with a healthy reproductive system.

As we grow up, we absorb a lot from our environment; most of it helps us to develop the tools that help us to function in the adult world. At the same time, a group of cells located in the back of our mind develops. This group of epigenetic cells absorbs emotions and memories of life, dealing with sometimes traumatic external or environmental factors. Many experiences and events in life can trigger emotional blockages in these cells. Some may be one time events, while others may be repeated events; some can be hidden traumas created from "normal parental behavior" or from environment behavior. Epigenetic cells cover some of our DNA and can make us think and make decisions from our fears hidden in them, rather than from the strong, emotional part of our DNA.

Go to the mirror, look at yourself and say: "I deserve…"

Take the first step: the step to serve only yourself, the step that will lead you to a happy future, a future centered on your own family… the children you proudly brought into the world in the most natural, exhilarating way.

Dr. Tzachi Topelberg

STRESSFUL LIFE AND HEALTH

For many years, the connection between stress and disease was a puzzle. The medical world was developing medicines for different diseases, while the mental health world developed tools for mental health.

During the last century, the understanding between stress and illness evolved to the point of agreement that there is a direct connection between them. In the last ten years, the medical world has admitted that many illnesses previously connected to elements like DNA, food and the environment, are also connected to a patient's stress levels and mental state.

During my years of practice, I have encountered two types of illness connected to stress: one is phantom pain, and the other is physical illness with a direct connection to mental state during stress.

The following are descriptions of people whom I treated, finding a relationship between their mental state and the physical illness they suffered from.

PHANTOM PAIN

Eighteen-year-old male high school student. He arrived for therapy due to problems at school, mainly low grades and misbehaving, along with anger toward the world. Along with that, he wanted to join the military and become a combat soldier. In order to get in shape, he was training with a paramilitary group that trains young people in physical and mental military skills.

During the first therapy session, I noticed that, every few minutes, he touched the back of his neck above the shoulders. When I asked him why, he told me that he suffered from a disc problem. However, he had never been positively diagnosed for such problem. The other thing he complained about was an old stress fracture in his left foot. He told me that during training, when he needed to sprint or undertake long marches, the pain in his foot intensified to the point where he needed to stop and would be unable to finish the exercise.

As the therapy process developed, I found that he suffered from fear of failure and low self-esteem. His parents were divorced, both M.D's. His mother had been protective and controlling from birth, while his father was both physically and mentally aggressive. A big portion of this man's exchanges with his son was to tell him that he was worth nothing. The results were reflected in the boy's bad behavior, depression and rapid ejaculation during sex. His fear of how he was perceived by his environment led him principally to fail; i.e. rather than try to do his utmost to succeed, instead, he would fail in advance, using many excuses, blaming his surrounding environment.

Without going into the whole therapy process here, I noticed that during the therapy, he complained less about his neck and his foot; I told him that, in my view, his pain was based on an inner brain process, and not a reflection of a physical trauma.

He presently joined the military and went to Special Forces evaluation. The military evaluation involved a lot of physical effort, along with mental evaluation. At first, he complained about his foot, then about his neck. He was sent by the military for MRI scans and X-rays to his neck and his foot. The results were negative in both cases; he was found to be healthy, with no physical trauma. He was not accepted into the Special Forces; moreover, he served a short service in a non-combat post.

We need to remember that DNA also has a part in mental healing. Courage is in our DNA. We cannot enhance our inner courage, which has a significant factor in the therapy process, challenging how far a person is willing to meet his or her fears and commence a dialog with them.

Our young operative is nineteen-and-a-half now, much better regarding his pain and much better in his sexual relationships. However, he has not quite managed yet to balance himself and remove stress to the point where it no longer drives his actions. He makes slow progress, and still chooses easy targets in order to avoid failure, when the results are not certain.

TRAUMA AND STRESS

Male, aged thirty-one, married for the second time; one child; a music teacher and performer. He stuttered badly, had very low self-esteem, and was stuck in a life of great ambition but with zero going on. At one time, he had attended speech therapy sessions, but after four months of treatment, he still stuttered as though he had received no treatment at all.

After a few meetings in which I analyzed and mapped his barriers, I began to understand the source of his problem. He was raised in a very religious environment; from primary school, his education had been very strict and demanding. Without elaborating about the way his parents raised him, I found another significant factor related to school: his tutor was not only a tough, intimidating person, but he also picked on him as a scapegoat and bullied him on a daily basis. The result was a deep fear of authority expressed in every aspect in his life. He considered the world surrounding him threatening and the feeling of rejection was controlling him. A further trauma had occurred at the age of eleven: an adult lured him in broad daylight from a safe, crowded place. The boy's need to feel important was the reason he allowed himself to be drawn into danger. The adult lured him to the entrance of a building and into the staircase area, then tried to attack him sexually. He recovered himself, and very bravely fled the place before the man succeeded in causing any lasting harm.

Since he was married, did not have any apparent sexual problems, and had a son, I needed to place every trauma in the correct proportion in order to continue the therapy process. I determined that the sexual attack played a secondary impact, and the teacher was his major trauma.

As I mentioned, he was brave. He was willing to collaborate with any task I gave him. He did not have any physical problem with his mouth or tongue. The treatment was conducted on two levels. The first was a dialogue with me to enable my diagnosis of the damage inflicted to his epigenetic area as a child, and to agree the problem and the inner dialogue with his fears. The other direction was to give him tasks in the outside world. These included approaching people he did not know with questions, calling music editors and music agents he did not know in order to set appointments and trying to promote his music.

The process took about six months. By this time, he had started to stabilize himself economically, his stutter was reduced to few syllables and after two more months, he no longer stuttered at all.

As we see in the above story, trauma and stress can cause physical and mental health problems. There is no knowing how trauma or stress will affect our health. The main thing is to show that, just as the brain can inflict illness, it can also heal illness if we know how to eliminate the trauma or the stress in such a way that we identify it, but use it to handle the trauma and the stress.

STRESS

Twins, seventeen years old. At the age of sixteen, both went to a life coach. During the course, one left due to maltreatment and offensive words from the coach, accusing him of lessening his twin. The other twin left shortly after, and when he came to see me for the first time, his mental state was very low. Both brothers suffered from Juvenile Myoclonic Epilepsy (JME). One of the brothers had recuperated from epilepsy, while the one that came for treatment was still suffering from it. Medical tests had found that their seizures occurred mainly in two circumstances: sleep deprivation and stress. Both brothers were being treated medically, and one was still taking medicine.

Raising twins is a big issue. Much research has been conducted regarding the raising of twins and how they grow up. A common agreement is that the best way to raise twins is to impose separation, starting from kindergarten. The purpose is to allow each to develop his own personality without the burden of an emotional connection while they are together among other children. Our twins went to the same school, but to different classes. Still, they went together to school, mingled with the same students during recess, and of course, returned to the same house carrying the same experiences daily.

When he arrived, I saw an introverted person who spoke very quietly, and had a very self-protective body language. His epilepsy manifested as mental freezing, with fixed eyes and detachment from his surroundings. He was on the proper medication; however, he still suffered seizures every two or three weeks. If he experienced a tense situation, the seizures happened more often and more strongly. At our first meeting, he froze up twice, his eyes fixed and with no awareness of what I'd said. Each freeze lasted about fifteen seconds.

During the therapy process, two main things emerged: a very caring mother, resulting in controlling tendencies. The other was much stronger - his brother. Although his brother did not do anything to belittle him, he felt that his brother was more successful, more socially accepted and, most significantly, no longer suffered from epilepsy.

As a result, he developed very low self-esteem. He was actually blocked from his surroundings and functioned automatically. He went to school, but had only one friend.

During school breaks, he stayed in class or stood by himself. He went out with his brother and friend, and although he was there, he acted as if he was not, not involving himself in any conversations, always 100% a follower. The twins went to practice basketball at a club. His always felt that his brother was more successful than he was.

After I revealed the series of events that had led him to this situation, I started the empowerment process. As in every therapy process, the patient usually has his defense mechanism ready... a set of excuses. Now his courage had to emerge. How strong would his will be to execute the tasks I gave him?

When he arrived, he was no longer playing basketball. I sent him to a boxing club, and he started Thai boxing. The most important was that he went there by himself, without his brother. Then I gave him more tasks to complete by himself. At one point, a girl from his school wanted to set him up with a date. Even though he told me that he was practically shaking with anxiety over this, I advised him to go along with the date - his first date ever. When I saw him next time, his body language was different, though he told me that he hadn't liked her. She was good looking enough, but played with her cell phone most of the time. He was bored, and since he was an intelligent person looking for conversation, he chose not to see her again. The punchline was that the girl who set up the date was, herself, interested in him. He said that he did not like her. This was a very significant stage in the therapy process. I asked him to show me her picture and tell me about her. I saw a pretty girl; he told me she was a smiler and a talker. To me, it jumped out that now was the moment to break his glass ceiling and come to the point of no return – meaning that if he crossed this bridge, he would never return to the box he'd lived in all his life. They are now a couple. It is moving slowly, but he is there. He is dating her; he is not being dragged along with friends to do nothing. He is slowly coming to terms with making their relationship public, and he is now in the fast lane.

So, why am I telling you this story?

For eight months now, he has suffered zero seizures. His grades are better, his understanding of himself is better, and I suggested that, since he liked to cook, he could prepare dinner for his family (his parents, two brothers and a sister). He agreed, and he did it. As his stress did not control him any longer, his body and mind became stronger. We await the one-year finish line, and if he is seizure-free for four more months, he will be medically approved as non-epileptic.

CONCLUSIONS

Stress has the ability to harm us physically. It can be a phantom pain, pain in our shoulders, back pains, indigestion problems, skin problems or one of many more "visible" medical problems. When we do not address the stress issues and keep on repressing them, the mind does not give up. If you do not pay attention to the warning signs you receive, the stress will intensify and the warning signs will be more significant. Each of us has different DNA. Each of us was raised differently, in different environments. Each of us looks at life events, and experiences them differently from others, even if both are in the same place. It is exactly like the known fact that if two people look at red paint, both will say they see red paint, yet each of them sees a different red paint. It is the same with stress. Every person has a unique stress. Stress based on the same characteristics can vary from person to person. Thus, the effects of stress will vary from person to person.

The inability to conceive can be one of the different medical problems that stress inflicts. A healthy reproductive system containing eggs with no pathological problem, and yet conception does not take place, is the result of a stress based on various anxieties. When a woman is undergoing IVF, she is actually an external tool expressing the stress; that is why the success rate of IVF is so low.

The correct way is to be brave, face your anxieties, acknowledge them, agree to their existence, cooperate with them instead of suppressing and ignoring them, and your level of stress will decrease. When you reduce the stress that prevents you from conceiving, it will be only a matter of a time before you are pregnant.

Before agreeing to hormone injections, expensive medical treatments and tense anticipation, be brave, look inside yourself, see how strong you are and fulfill your dream.

FEARING YOUR SPOUSE

The doorbell rang. I opened the door. She stood there, embarrassed and hesitant. I invited her in. Two days earlier, she had called me. "Dr. Topelberg, my name's Maya… a friend recommended I call you. I was a bit skeptical - after all, I'm a healthy woman, my husband's sperm count is balanced, and yet, five IVF procedures, and nothing's happened. Three years married, and I can't conceive…"

We set an appointment. I asked her to come alone. I always set the first appointment with the woman first… and there are reasons.

As with every case concerning issues of pregnancy, I always start with questions regarding the spousal relationship. This was a tough case.

There are many reasons why we connect to another human being to be married. One major obstacle is the dream we have when we are still single, and the picture of our spouse we paint in our mind.

There are two major characteristics regarding the interrelationship between a man and a woman when couples do not succeed in having a baby.

The first one is the dream of a tall, masculine man, very good looking and physically appealing. The problem in some of those cases of failure to conceive is that this macho man has very low self-esteem. He hides behind a manly job and manly walls, transmitting to the world the message: I am perfect. Well, he may not be. Moreover, he will be polite and helpful to other people, at work or with friends. However, within the relationship, he may be impatient, indecisive, and indifferent to the woman's needs. He can have angry outbursts and behave in a violent way, expressed mostly verbally.

A woman's dream of marrying a "man's man" often

rests on the need to be protected, to have a secure place in his strong arms. She loves the flattering feeling that she is a worthy woman since such a stud is interested in her. She likes the idea of her family and friends seeing her with such a handsome man. She knows that she is attractive, but depends on seduction, leading her away from confidence in her own ability to succeed in life. She is led by emotion mainly generated from lack of confidence, generated from low self-esteem. Her cognitive area is busy with, "How do I look?" and not with the best way to conduct a balanced relationship based on strong and understandable foundations. She expects him to lead, and finds herself struggling with daily decisions concerning herself and both of them. Her response will usually be to placate her spouse; all she wants is peace and quiet, a normal loving relationship, the ability to have constructive dialogue with him, and the ability to say anything without meeting a brick wall.

This comes from two main reasons: fear of abandonment, and fear of his reaction. Fear of abandonment in this case sits on two chairs: the first is that, regardless of his behavior, he is her idol and she is afraid that she will never find a physically attractive man like him again. Her dependency on this relationship chains her to him. The other is fear of his reaction... the words he might say, the punishment he might inflict (such as: not talking to her, or going out by himself for hours) and/or a verbal or physical punishment. She finds herself living under stress. She has her tender, good moments with him, and most probably good sex, followed by an emotional crash a moment later - the stress created from the emotional rollercoaster she experiences.

Stressful outcomes will result in various negative physical phenomena.

So, why doesn't she conceive?

She is a healthy woman! The main thing is what is happening in the back of her mind... the reasons that brought her to marry this type of man. She is in daily conflict. On one hand, she does not want to leave him, but on the other hand, she lives under stress and with low self-esteem, and now all those disturbing thoughts are sitting in the back of her mind and creating fear of what will happen when she has a baby. Will he abuse the baby as he abuses her? Will he support her after the labor and all through the stages of the child's development? She may also fear that the child will be like her spouse - violent and hurtful. One troubling fear is related to his possible abandonment of her and her child if she becomes no longer attractive to him. The troubling thought in the back of her mind is stopping her from conceiving.

We can barely distinguish between the thoughts we have in our cognitive area; we neither know, nor distinguish, the thoughts we have in the back of our brain. She needs to solve the stressful situation between her and her spouse. She needs to agree that she, too, needs to contribute to the healing process with her spouse.

If real love exists - not fearful love - and if sincere emotions are there, she will succeed. They both need to agree on a set of tools, which may help to turn down the heat and create a good dialog: send each other text messages during the day, and even if there's no immediate reply, it's okay, she's said what she wanted, and that's all that matters; make phone calls only if it's a matter of urgency. If he shouts, she should not reply, but should calmly say once what she wants, but back off if he continues to shout. If he refuses to listen to what she has to say, then she can write it down. She shouldn't be afraid to express what she wants, what she misses and what makes her feel good. If she doesn't hear the words "I love you," if she needs to implore him time after time to go out with him, to go out for a coffee together once a week, or go to a restaurant - now is the time for him to listen and let her lead. She needs to understand that the lack of communication, her fears and frustrations, and her fear of being abandoned will prevent her conceiving.

Should the situation not change, nothing will happen. If she agrees to lead, to say what she has in mind, to lead him to a communicative state of mind rather than a defensive state of mind, there will be huge smiles nine months later.

The second case is usually a woman married to a good hearted man who suffers from low self-esteem in his masculinity, though not necessarily at work, where he may be successful. The woman will be average, not glamorous, what the general population would consider to be an average looking person. The man feels, in a way, lucky that he's found a spouse. He will treat his spouse with respect, flatter her and let her take the lead. The problem may be that she does not want to lead. She likes the flattery and the respect; however, let us remember that she has low self-esteem regarding her looks or femininity. What she really wants is a dominant man in bed, helping her to feel better about her body, a man who helps her to open up sexually. Again, let us remember that he has low masculine self-esteem and is happy just to be having sex with a woman, and not wishing to be sexually dominant. It becomes a magic circle of the queen who does not want to rule.

So, why doesn't she conceive? The reason comes directly from her childhood, the relationship with her parents, brothers and sisters, and school. Somewhere along the trail of her childhood, between babyhood and the age of fifteen, a low self-esteem and lack of confidence developed in her. She definitely missed hugs and attention, and felt insecure in her body, and the man she met allegedly fills all those needs. Still, her fear of failure is stronger than the compliments she receives, and her low self-esteem completes the barrier preventing her from becoming pregnant.

What can she do? There are many exercises to upgrade self-esteem. First, she needs to accept her body, be able to stand nude in front of a full size mirror, look at her body and understand that this body was given to her, like it or not, and it will remain. If her man is not a leader during sex, she could find a fantasy that she likes, and ask him to act it out with her. If she experiences constant self-pity, she needs to remember that no one will do for her what she can do for herself, and what happened in the past remains there… she needs to be a strong, adult person and not a rejected kid. One big obstacle is the release of control in front of her spouse; releasing control is something she deserves to enjoy. She should tell her spouse, next time they have sex, how she would like to start it, perhaps with her on her back, arms and legs spread, eyes covered… and he should delight her. She shouldn't attend to his needs, but allow herself to focus only on her own pleasure.

There should be a time limit. If they both make progress in the relationship, then they are going the right way; however, if the old patterns of behavior keep cropping up, perhaps she should think again about what is keeping her with this person. She should avoid thinking about what she will lose if she leaves him, but think what she'll gain. Keeping on hoping for the word "if" will waste time she can never recover.

And what happened with Maya? Her husband agreed to start seeing me, and went through an anger prevention therapy process. During the process, he understood that his anger came from other places and Maya was merely an easy target when his frustration, leading to anger, overcame him. Maya, on the other hand, learned two main things: not to be dragged into an argument, but reply quietly on the spot or at a later, appropriate time; and during sex, she learned to ask for her desires rather than to just satisfy her husband to show him how good she is. A therapy process cannot alter the mind instantly. After we understand, agree, and try to act differently, our minds take time to adjust. However, when I perform a pregnancy therapy process, the main target is opening the blocked channel for pregnancy. In this case, the biggest issue was trust. At the end of the process, which took three months, Maya conceived and received her beautiful gift nine months later. She was called Tanya, after my initials, to my great pleasure.

LOW SELF-ESTEEM

She came through the door, and honestly, I am a man of the world, but I lost my breath for a moment. She was 5ft 7in tall, with beautiful, long curly hair and a painted, beautiful, feminine face. By the time ten minutes had passed, I learned that she had three B.A. and two M.A. degrees, all in different professions. She was forty-three years of age, single and in a high ranked government position. She spoke very quickly; it took me a few minutes to elicit the following: she had frozen some eggs, she did not have a spouse, and she suffered from fibromyalgia.[*]

She had undergone IVF twice with no success, and she still had four eggs in deep freeze. I tried to catch up with her speed-of light-thoughts and speech. It took a while, and by the time she slowed down and relaxed a little, I also understood she had her last relationship not long ago; the man was famous, rich, single, good looking, forty years of age, a courting type who gave her everything… and she left him.

Imagine yourself on an island, survivor of a storm that wrecked your boat. The sand is white and the beautiful coconut trees give shade. Your clothes are ragged, and you have no water and no food. Suddenly it rains so heavily that you hunch up under a tree, feeling miserable and sorry for yourself, wondering what will happen to you. Now imagine you have landed on that same island and you start to explore the area, and just behind a small hill, two miles from your landing point, you find a village with hospitable people, food, water and means of communicating with the world.

It makes no difference if you are very intelligent or not,

[*] https://en.wikipedia.org/wiki/Fibromyalgia

very pretty or not, poor or rich... low self-esteem is the gap between your real abilities and what you *think* your abilities are. Low self-esteem can appear in many forms: the inability to have a friend, settling for a reasonably paid job but nothing more... or one can be a CEO and still be unable to conceive. The blockage in the mind that prevents conception is connected to other effects emerging from low self-esteem, but does not necessarily affect every aspect of life.

Low self-esteem is usually connected to the mother-daughter relationship. Of course, a strong father can have an affect directly or indirectly, in school and in the neighborhood. In general, the way we grow and develop is strongly connected to our parents; however, our subject is babies, so I shall stick to that.

Despite the fact that she loves your body, enjoys sex and has no problem attaining an orgasm, conceiving a baby still eludes her? Fear of failure is the main cause. It reflects like a spider's web on a variety of subjects. It is her self-concept regarding how others see her. She tries to prove herself at work, she tries to be innovative and think outside the box... at work. She will be pleasant and cooperative... at work. This may lead her to try to find a very successful man, good looking and, most importantly, flattering to her being. Now she has a spouse, a job, and her life is an object of envy to the world.

However, obsessive thinking in the back of the mind will not stop these questions: what happens if he stops loving me? Or leaves me? Or if I can't be as successful at having a baby and being a mother as I have been in everything else? There is a long way to fall.

Women suffering from low self-esteem will mostly have male friends, or a male best friend, rather than a female best friend. The reason for this is twofold: firstly, there is no intimate obligation to the male friend, hence she does not suffer any tension or stress, and while he may desire her, he won't tell her, while she, on the other hand, enjoys his cooperation as a friend, his company, or his willingness to help out with odd jobs and chat on the phone, while a female friend can be a source of tension; the other reason is that there is no competition. A close female friend may be on the same level of life as her... however, that friend may have a good relationship, be married or possibly pregnant, with stability in her life, and there may also be jealousy over looks, success and more. This can lead to this thought: every time I am with her I feel like shrinking because she has achieved what I want to achieve but haven't yet succeeded in.

Low self-esteem can bring additional anxieties: what happens if she becomes pregnant and is all by herself, with no spouse or family to support her? And what about the need for freedom regarding her career?

In terms of career, there are two issues: one is the need to prove how worthy she is – the need for the people at work to appreciate her ability to be really good at what she does, and even more, to be above average. Outstanding, even! This attitude will bring her the compliments she needs; she aspires to have all that in order to be reassured that she is worthy. The problem is that she needs to go through this process every day. Every day, when she wakes up and gets organized for a new day, the list of troubling thoughts escorts her as she dresses, puts on her makeup and makes her way to work. She almost feels like the shepherd filling the trough with water so that her sheep will be grateful and will show it by following her as a leader, while the truth is that she expects her sheep to give her wool.

The other issue is financial security. When she thinks of a baby in her arms, she feels excitement and joy, but at the same time she is filled with the worry that she will not be able to give the baby a good enough life because now, she cannot continue with her career. The thought that she is not good enough leaps out from the back of her mind, controlling her, and finds a way out by creating excuses reflected by her, the grown-up who is being managed by a scared child.

The inner dialogue she can create with herself is a key factor to removing blocking thoughts. Failure needs to be a jumping-off point, not a blocking point. Thinking about what she is afraid of and endless vague possibilities will provide no benefit; thinking of what is in her hands and within her power will fulfill what she wants.

So what can she do?

First, she must understand that what others think of her has no relevance to who she really is. If she could see a movie showing her other people's lives, she would be amazed to see how stressful the world of those people she looks up to actually is. She needs to understand that some people around her are motivated by envy, lack of confidence, low self-esteem and more. She even may find herself being hurt by them... they may try to fail her on purpose, talk behind her back, or gossip. All of that is because she is a successful person, with enviable talents. She is the strong one, not they. She must understand that all of that comes from their weaknesses and not because they are better than she is.

She should find a place in her life that makes her a little afraid: ask her partner to blindfold her during sex, go on a roller coaster, put on a bikini and go by herself to the beach or pool, or take a bus to someplace unknown to her, without her cell phone, and wander around taking in the sights, go shopping, have a coffee... and do it for a couple of hours. When she's done, she should ask directions to the bus station, remembering that she must be far from the station and have no knowledge of where the station is. Maybe she should go out without any makeup on, or find some place in her life she usually avoids, and go there. She will realize that nothing bad will happen, even if she does it again in the same place or in another scary place. Initially, she should choose the less scary places, and only go to the more difficult places later on. She will see very quickly that she has agreed to allow herself to be afraid; at this point, her fears will start to dissolve, since when we address a fear, it is not frightening anymore. Regardless of her qualifications, she needs to agree with herself that she is willing to be unworthy. This way, she will no longer expect judgment from her surroundings. Agreeing to be unworthy does not mean dismissing herself from the world surrounding her. It means that she understands herself and requires no confirmation from the world about her qualifications, her abilities or her looks.

What about the beginning of our story? The curly-haired woman? Her age did not allow me to conduct a long therapy process; I needed to find the exact spot in her mind preventing her from conceiving. The meetings were very quick and I admit that I gave her a difficult time by reflecting upon her the barriers stopping her from conceiving. Yet, at the same time, I reflected to her the strong and powerful woman she was. She learned that she had inflicted sorrow only on herself. She learned to differentiate between things she had control over and things outside her control. After four meetings she went through IVF again… and she now has twins. She did not quit her job. When the twins were a year old, she found a husband, a divorced man of fifty with two children of his own. They are now planning a child together.

Imagine you are alone on an island. No one can tell you anything because there is no one there but you. It is your choice, to sit, do nothing, full of despair and feel sorry for yourself, hoping that someone will rescue you.

Your other option is to decide to survive - no matter what you thought of yourself before, no matter what you think people have said about you, no matter how low your self-esteem. If you decide to live, you will find inside yourself powers and abilities you never knew were there. Define all your negative thoughts, decide to live and decide what is driving you. When you stop hiding, you will no longer need anyone telling you how great you are. You will be the one to show the world how great you are, because now you know.

MOMMY ISSUES

Blond, blue eyes and fair skin... mmm... and a crumpled face as she walked into my clinic. The nervous movements of her face testified to the stress and distress she was in.

Olga was thirty-two, and had been living with her husband for two years. The main reason leading her to come was troubling thoughts concerning fear of abandonment. During our first meeting, I heard many examples such as: "I send a text message to my husband and if he doesn't return them promptly, I've a feeling he wants to leave me," or "If he says he's going to meet a friend straight from work, it tells me he doesn't want to be with me." The fact that not all signs from him indicated that he wanted to be apart from her failed to stop these troubling thoughts. The same had occurred to Olga - with friends, at work, and all through her life. When we discussed her sexuality, she told me that she enjoyed sex. However, when we elaborated, it appeared that Olga liked to delight her spouse, but she had never asked any sexual partner to delight her.

IMPORTANT:

MOTHERS DO EVERYTHING FROM LOVE. ANY DAMAGE INFLICTED ON YOU IS UNINTENTIONAL AND COMES FROM LACK OF KNOWLEDGE AND LACK OF SELF EVALUATION.

MOTHERS WANT ONLY THE BEST FOR THEIR CHILDREN.

After understanding the big picture, I asked Olga one question: what is the nature of your relationship with your mother?

And all hell broke loose! To be continued...

There is no doubt that most of you love your mother. Mothers come in many shapes and forms; they can be homemakers or executives, single mothers or married. Well, this is a narrow aspect of the person and constitutes only a minor part of your mother-daughter relationship. Now let's talk of the conversation your mother has had with you, the conversation that started when you were a baby and went on... well, sometimes, till today.

The first mother model is the caring mother, the mother who protects you the entire day, day after day. She will constantly make sure you're okay and that you have everything you need. Should you have any difficulty, say in school, a tutor will be assigned for you... she provides your favorite food, clothing, and all the comfort you need. Along with this wonderful care, she will always try to strengthen you, tell you how talented you are, how beautiful you are, and that you deserve all the best in the world because you are so wonderful. She will protect you from your surroundings, preventing you from failure in any respect, even in sister/brother or father/daughter relationships.

All in all, you may grow up as a very normal person, have a happy childhood, and - usually - your grades at school will not be straight As. This will become clear later, only after you go through a therapy process and reveal what a strong, clever person you really are. No one can look at a child and guess how he will be in adulthood; there endless variants gathering along the way, shaping the mind of a person. However, our subject matter today is pregnancy.

The result of our mother/daughter relationship is hidden in the back of your mind. On the one hand, you have very good relationship with your mother, and you may consider her to be your best friend. Due to her overprotective attitude, you develop a hidden fear of failing, coming directly from the fact that you almost never failed. A failure is: a choice I make, it depends only on me, I do my utmost to succeed… and I do not.

Now. A fear of failure is a fear of success. Why? It isn't that I don't want to succeed, but for success, I need that, at the end, success will be promised to me. In other words, tell me the end result before I even start. Of course, no one can tell you the end. In parallel, you do not want to fail or admit failure. Remember the protective process you had as a child, creating the fear of failure. What is your solution now? Create excuses, avoid decisions, and by doing so, you avoid hearing the words "You failed" since you have the ready-made excuse: "I already told you I've no interest in doing that… it's stupid… I've no desire to learn this because the teaching level there is so poor… there's no demand for this profession…" The list of excuses is endless. Now, in terms of your emotions, you develop a fear of abandonment connected to your fear of failure. This hides really deep in the back of your mind. Your cognitive area has no idea or any notion, however, when what crosses your mind is that if you fail, how will your mother react? Or rather, how will you face her after you fail? It's not just the baby - it's how will the baby be? How will he grow? And so on. This fear of failure creates a subconscious blockage that prevents conception and pregnancy.

So, what can you do?

Well, let us define failure first. It is a choice you make, depending only on you, when you do your utmost to reach the target, but you do not succeed. There is a difference between a "mistake" and "failure." Go to a bar by yourself, let a man approach you, and if one appeals to you, allow him to sit with you and have a nice conversation. But in the end, you will not give him your phone number. If you are married, do something you are not good at. Perhaps if you do not cook, then do it. If you cannot decide on a vacation? Go, learn to face the places you are afraid to visit and go there.

And what of your mother? It depends. She might call you a few times a day - or, if you do not call her, she gets insulted. When you talk, perhaps she gives you advice that you do not want to hear, or criticizes your lifestyle. Yes, keep in touch with your mother, but, give her less information about your life. Do not elaborate. If she criticizes, let her talk, do not argue, do not be insulted. Keep your contact with her as a loving mother and not as a consultant. Once you overcome your fear of failing, you will not be aggravated by your mother any more. Once you understand that *you* run your life and failure is part of your development as a person... then a baby will soon come.

The second mother type is the boss /teacher / commander. She will tell you, from the first day you remember, what is best for you. She will have an opinion when you tell her anything, even if it is not a question. She will correct you, advise you, and be insulted if you refuse to listen to her.

Since this type of relationship goes on practically from your birth, a negative connotation is being created in your mind. On the one hand, you love your mother, but on the other hand, you are snappy and jumpy when she talks to you. What happens in your mind is actually dependency and desperation anxiety. In a way, you wait for these calls or conversations since you suffer from fear of success. This fear of success is projected as dependency on your mother; you wait for these conversations like a drug addict. You take your fears and throw them at your mother by allowing yourself to submit to your anger at her control over you. You may not be surprised when I suggest that you have difficulty making decisions. In the back of your mind, the anxiety over what your mother will tell you about your decisions prevents you from even taking any decisions, and the thought of your mother's eternal intervention from the moment you conceive freezes your body and prevents you from getting pregnant.

So, what can you do?

Yes, do talk to your mother. However, tell her as little as possible about your life - do not hide, but do not elaborate. When she gives you her speeches, remarks and opinions, just listen. Yes, it is very difficult, but this is the first step to freeing yourself. In the beginning, just say that all is well, work is okay, and your husband is okay - without elaborating. It is not simple. She does not need to know what you did last night, or which friends you visited at the weekend. Again, if you do tell, whatever your mother has to say should not evolve into a conversation that will lead to criticism that irritates you as it has done up till this point. Arguing serves two purposes: the first is that it supplies the fuel for the other person who likes to argue (the more you disagree, the more she will argue); the other thing is that when you argue with your mother, you agree to run from facing yourself, avoiding things in you that stop you. In a hidden way, when you argue with your mother, you expect her to give you a solution, but in fact, you know that her solution is not good for you. Learn to take responsibility for your decisions and you will no longer feel the need to argue with your mother. It is not simple to go through such a process. Develop a vacuum inside yourself. Now you have nowhere to run with your fears. Now, you need to have a self-dialogue. This is the beginning of facing yourself, your fears, and a moment later, you face the fact that you are strong, you can decide, you are afraid, but it is not stopping you, and a moment later, before you fully understand the brave process you went through, you are pregnant.

As I mentioned at the beginning, a mother's behavior and its effect on children comes in many variations. I have encountered this phenomenon often during years of therapy. However, one thing is salient, and many of the women I treated concerning pregnancy issues had a dependency on their mother, be it positive or negative. If you are healthy and your life is stable, but in this entire situation, the only thing that emerges is a tension from or toward your mother, then this is the reason you do not conceive and, if this issue is solved, you will get pregnant.

Olga could not stop her tears. It was a while before she could answer my questions. Olga's mother was a bossy woman; she actually treated Olga like a programmable robot. She used to tell her what should she do, what to wear, criticize her friends, and phrases like, "You could do better," were common. And as Olga grew up and left home, there were the phone conversations... her mother's control of her never ceased. What Olga developed was a fear of her mother's authority; this fear had developed into a fear of failure.

Olga felt that in her everyday life, people were looking at her and judging her. She became insecure to the point where she couldn't have an orgasm. Always, when she was sexually aroused, she shut down a second before the orgasm. I found that she felt unworthy, but she did not deserve to feel this. Olga had to overcome this obstacle by telling herself that if she wanted something, she deserved it, only for herself. All of those anxieties concentrated to become one significant fear: what will happen if my pregnancy does not go well, or if the baby is not okay?

Part of the therapy process was to give Olga the tools teaching her to release control. What it actually meant was leading her to agree to go along with a fear so as to not be blocked by fears.

Olga also reduced the communication with her mother to basic information about her life. She learned not to be aggravated by things her mother said. Olga learned to conduct a self-dialogue and to understand her strong points; she understood that to release control is to actually be in full control of your strong points and not be controlled by your fears.

Olga has not yet learned to have an orgasm, perhaps because she is now in the sixteenth week of her pregnancy.

FEARING THE WORLD

Many people in the world suffer from different phobias concerning the world we live in. In this chapter, I will elaborate how phobias prevent pregnancy.

Jasmin was thirty-two when she came for our first meeting. She had been married for three years, had a good job, a nice house, and from the outside she and her husband were just a normal married couple. Soon I found that what lead Jasmin through her everyday life was the question: "What if…?" On the one hand, she had neither OCD, nor disturbing pathological thoughts. She was an intelligent, confident and assertive person. What she could tell me was that during a normal day, if she heard a news flash about a bomb anywhere in the world, her body would contract and she would be flooded with the horror that, at the end of her working day, when she was about to leave the building, it would happen to her. Jasmin's fears lay in every event or even the speculation of an event. For instance, if there was a tsunami somewhere two years ago, the fear of a tsunami would escort her even near a calm pond. Slowly, her fears became more vague, and she started to feel a less defined fear that something bad would happen without being able to pinpoint anything specific, just a feeling of fear in general.

Fear of the world can prevent a woman from conducting a normal life. It may be a fear of violence, of a car accident, the weather or one of many things her mind decides is a threat. She may avoid doing particular things or being in certain places. However, the fear she is aware of is just a fraction of what is happening in the back of her mind. So, now let us connect the fear to motherly emotion. There is a difference between being afraid for herself and being afraid for her unborn child.

As for us, we can go to seminars, discuss the hand of

fate in a human life, and have a big hug if we are afraid. Those tools allow us to somewhat calm our fears about the destruction of the Earth or any other catastrophe. Now, remember this fact: you do have worries and anxieties about bad things happening in the world, and due to supportive surroundings, you manage to conduct a balanced life, but in the back of your mind, no one hugs you. Your fears will not necessarily emerge as a big catastrophe every day. You start to develop mistrust. If you need a handyman, or if you buy a car, you may debate with yourself, ask others and have difficulty reaching a decision, not because you are a hesitant person, but because you do not trust. As I mentioned above, a woman's motherly instinct and her will to become a mother plays an important role. The process in the back of her mind creates some harrowing pictures of the world into which her child will be born; starting from his health as an infant, she then imagines how risky a place school can be - the stairs, the campus, exposure to childhood diseases – and what will happen when he or she lives by himself or herself when they go to college and on? All she wants to do is to protect her child, but since this child is not yet born, there is one way she can be sure to protect him a hundred percent.

So, what can she do?

If constant anxieties prevent a person from conducting a balanced life, one way is to see a psychiatrist and obtain a prescription for antidepressants. Whatever medication is recommended, know that it is only helping the patient through the balancing process; they will not necessarily have to continue taking any medicine. Anti-anxiety medicines should be taken alongside cognitive therapy.

The next step is for the patient to understand their very deep fear of failure; the fear is actually using the risks existing in the world to make the patient hide and prevent their self-fulfillment - and pregnancy. In order to break the glass ceiling from fear of failure, it is necessary to think of one or more situations, including sexual situations that engender fear. The principle is to make a decision: take a piece of paper and divide it into two columns, one for benefits, and the other for what happens if you are wrong. From the moment the decision is made that you want to buy or do something, allow no more than three days to pass before you do it. (I do not mean significant, life-changing actions like buying a house or relocation.)

As the decision is made, imagine walking toward the "mistake" column, but do your utmost to achieve the other column. Visualize one or more such situations. The realization soon comes that you are not dead; nothing bad happened to you. If you were mistaken, you can learn for the next time and not become a victim of yourself. Now, you are on the right track to be able to conceive the natural way and to understand that you cannot control the world, but you should enjoy the good the world has to offer.

Back to Jasmin. She had a dream of how her family would look, a big house, money, status, and at the same time her mother was "helping" her by telling her how her life should look and what should she do. Jasmin took 5mg Cipralex daily, stopping it after five weeks. She was now able to concentrate on our meetings and the tasks I gave her.

It is never easy to touch fears. If I gave her a task, I, as her therapist, was not really concerned if she fulfilled the task a hundred percent. For me, her agreement to try the task and her willingness to perform the task testified to a positive process already starting in the back of her mind. The discussion of her task results, the feelings she experienced and her new insights, enabled her to approach the next task better placed. As she was experiencing new things, a positive process was intensifying in her brain. Remember, our process was to try and pinpoint the blocked mental channel preventing her from conceiving.

It took me a weekly meeting for three months to lead Jasmin toward balanced thinking. Why three months?

Because she conceived after ten weeks' treatment. In the twelfth, she found out she was pregnant and we stopped. We agreed that after the baby was born, she would come again to continue her therapy in order to enable her better, balanced life.

Fears have a tendency to grow and influence us even more strongly in a negative way with the passage of time. The longer we wait to solve our fears, the harder it is to get rid of them.

The major factor holding us when we look at the world with fear is how we perceive death. The more we fear death, the more we prevent ourselves from living. No, we do not have to die in order to remove that fear; we need to not only understand it in a cognitive way, but also in the back of our minds. Since death is inevitable and we cannot control it, we need to free our minds and allow the world, the one we fear, to contain us. Try to ease control in your daily life, and develop trust in your surroundings. Do not try to control; relaxing yourself into the world will let you be a happy mother sooner that you imagine.

BABY HEALTH ISSUES

Many health parameters are checked before pregnancy: the parents' DNA match, the family history etc., to evaluate the potential for defects, both physical and mental, in the infant. During pregnancy, there are also many tests to check the embryo's health and development. Then there's labor and the associated risks. Yet, millions of healthy babies are born and grow up to have good, balanced and happy lives. Moreover, the rules about delivery and the tools of delivery have changed. Forceps delivery is out in many countries due to the harm it causes (mainly scalp damage) during labor. So, a woman is checked from before the pregnancy, throughout the pregnancy and is well taken care of during labor.

Daphne was thirty-four, a lawyer, and had been married for two years. At our first meeting, she told me that she had already undergone two rounds of IVF with no success. The field of her expertise was criminal law; I mention that because, later, I found a connection between her fears about the baby's health and her occupation.

The barrier in a woman's mind, when it comes to trouble conceiving due to anxiety about the baby's health, lies in two channels: the first affects an active woman – she loves life, she has an active career, she likes her vacations and lives the good life. When she sees, or encounters in any way, a woman handling a disabled child, her body contracts. The thought that her life could cease to exist as she knows it, transformed to nonstop caring for a disabled child, freezes her and the back of her mind creates harrowing options that, basically, instruct her body not to accept a pregnancy that could stop her joyful life. The other affects a sensitive, emotional woman, a very caring person who tries to make the world around her perfect. She is a person who likes to know everything, likes to help others and give advice. She is constantly anxious that all will be in good order and correct, i.e. she will not only want to know everything, but also want to fix things. This is a controlling person, not in a bad, aggressive way, but a *caring*, controlling person.

Both ladies should notify themselves that now is the time to ask why they are not getting pregnant.

When a woman has a baby, she actually agrees to lose control. If the baby gets sick (which is very normal for babies), she may develop deep stress, not about the normal 'flu the baby has, but about all the complications she has heard may result from the 'flu. She may become stressed about germs harming the baby even though she may not have any special issues regarding germs for herself.

It is common knowledge that the immune system develops better when the body is exposed to the environment. If you raise a baby in an isolated, clean environment, his immune system will not be able to learn how to attack infection or illness. Many autoimmune illnesses emerge at a young age from mental stress inflicted at home; it can be overprotection, or mistreatment.

Babies are strong; they can survive a high fever that would make a grown-up faint; they can fall and stay intact because their bones are soft. Babies are much stronger than we think. Just following medical advice on how to treat a baby will help him to grow up healthy.

What can you do?

First, a woman needs to check the genetic history of her family and her spouse's family, in order to learn of any hereditary diseases. This check is meant to eliminate the potential of known hereditary disorders or diseases affecting their child. Now she can be reassured that her future child will be born healthy.

During the pregnancy, she should follow medical advice and she will go through the pregnancy period balanced. And what of her fears? Indeed, a pregnant woman somehow influences the embryo by the food she eats, by her physical activity, by the stress she experiences. There is no exact science or indication of how a mother's behavior can affect the embryo.

After the birth, all she can do is help her child grow into life. She can provide tools, knowledge, warmth and love, but she cannot decide what her child will become as he grows. Remember, a child has her genes, her husband's genes and the genes of previous generations on both sides.

Should you overprotect your child, you may encourage traumas or phobias. Overprotection will develop a fear of failure in the child as he grows.

A mother must agree with herself that her child will get sick at times, and that this is actually good for him, as it will develop his immune system. She needs to allow in her mind that her child will fail, and that he is not there to fulfill her frustrated ambitions and unfulfilled wishes from her past.

And if the child has no genetic problems, please, mothers, do not inflict your fears on him. Allow yourself to be the proud, frightened mother of a mentally and physically healthy child.

Back to Daphne. First her husband: it appeared that he was good looking, but less successful than his wife. His emotional intelligence was low, and Daphne could not get proper, manly support from him in decisions regarding their life together, nor as a sex partner. Sex was okay, but Daphne, insecure with her body, needed a man who could give her confidence. I gave them both tasks related to their relationship, and to sex. Daphne's main issue was that she did not know to make demands for herself; she could not say, "I deserve…" This issue occurs in many life-blocking areas. The baby health issue was directly connected to her anxieties concerning herself. Amongst other issues was the fear that she would not be able to protect the baby's health and well-being. Daphne also had a fear concerning her husband, that she would not receive the proper support from him if something went wrong with the baby.

They needed an exercise that they would both benefit from: Daphne's husband needed to take control, and Daphne needed to release control. I told them that the next time they had sex, Daphne was to lie on her back, arms and legs spread, her eyes covered, and her husband should pamper her by following her instructions. Daphne was instructed not to touch her husband at all throughout the process.

I gave Daphne more tasks to make her understand that when the baby came, she could only provide care and treatment, but would not be able to determine when 'flu or rubella would decide to visit.

We worked on this matter and Daphne, after solving a few of her self-issues, together with her cooperative husband, got pregnant. When the baby was a year old, she got pregnant again. She told me that she wants now to make up for all the lost years she lived as a fugitive from this world.

KNOWING THE FUTURE

Remember, we as people cannot be in control of, or be responsible for other people, in such a way that we influence 100% of their lives. No one can sign off on what will happen in the end. The result is a sum of many random things that cannot be decided or guaranteed at the outset. The phenomenon regarding inability to conceive is directly related to this.

Aimee was thirty-eight, a good-looking girl. During our first session, I realized that Aimee was not very secure at work; she tended to discuss her superior from the standpoint of "I know better and the way the things are now is not the best way." After a few meetings, the main problem was identified: Aimee wanted to be sure of the outcome of any event or situation with which she was involved, and if she was not sure, she tended to try to make it sure. Insecurity controlled her totally.

How can we know what will happen in the end? When we meet a person, when we set off on a car journey, when we go to sleep, or meet with friends… the answer is that we cannot know the outcome in advance. Of course, we plan, we make estimates based on the information we have, and, indeed, things mainly end as we expected. However, this is only true for short-term events and events about which we have a lot of information in advance.

Conceiving is strongly influenced by a woman's constant need to know what will happen in the end. Because of that, making decisions is a problem for her and indecision takes over. Questions arise, such as: maybe the other option is better, or what will others say about my decision? However, at the same time a very argumentative person appears on the scene - a person fighting to prove that she is right.

What drives our anxieties are the experiences that

shaped our mind as children, together with our DNA.

With reference to pregnancy, uncertainty about a newborn baby can result in scrambled questions in the back of a woman's mind: Will he/she be born healthy? Will he develop properly, be smart, be physically capable, a good student? Will he find a girl good enough for him and have a happy, successful marriage? Will he be financially successful? Will he support me in my old age? Those thoughts do not dissipate and lie in front of her like a written document.

The issue "I need you to assure me of the final result of any decision" actually affects many phobias, especially as the sufferer will not believe anyone who tries to assure her. Those life-blocking phobias are reflected while looking for a job, finding a spouse, buying a car or television, and many more. All of them result quite often in just doing nothing. This phobia directly reflects fear of the future concerning loss of self-control, and prevents conception.

A woman should never forget that she is a worthy person and a worthy woman, that she is stronger than all her past influences, and that she *can* do it all. She can see her body as a functioning machine, set her mind free and let her healthy, ready-made biological system work and serve her for the purpose of fulfilling her birthright.

So, what can you do?

First, I want to emphasize that an outward lack of confidence is not necessarily connected to the inability to conceive.

When a woman is afraid to start things, she mostly avoids doing them at all. In order to break those barriers, she should try to be brave by doing new things, choosing small things to begin with, and then going for the more intimidating actions. This way, she will start to realize that, when she starts any new venture without knowing the results, the sky does not fall in. After her mind starts to relax because the fear of the results is fading, her body will be ready to conceive.

Go to a dance club, by yourself. Have fun, but return home by yourself, no matter whom you meet. If you fear roller-coasters – do it, by yourself. It's okay to tell a person standing in line or someone sitting near you in the car that you're afraid. Create something and show to your friend, agreeing to accept criticism. Go out without any makeup. Look at your life and measure how much you give to others compared to how much you give to yourself. Giving to yourself is not necessarily buying something - it's mainly using your power to fulfill your wishes. Examine how much you fear authority, mainly male authority. Write down your strong points, your weak points and compare them to what people say about you.

What of Aimee? She slowly opened up. She became willing to accept that things in her world - like her husband and her job - may end, but it would not mean the end of her world. Life can reemerge after loss. She was willing to conduct herself in a different way in regard to her intimate relationship with her husband, and to play a dominant part in their sexual activity, rather than just indulging him to show him how good she was. Her frustrations about herself and her life, and her fears about her surroundings, were reduced. It took four months of treatment. One night, or rather, one day, when she agreed to be submissive to her body, and to free her mind of questions and disturbing thoughts, she conceived; now Aimee has three children... and a husband.

She promised herself that she would raise her children in a different way, and learn the best way to avoid creating life blocking fears in her children.

Remember - the future is now.

Babyphobia

CAREER ISSUES

Equal opportunities for all, including women, feature large in our world today. Furthermore, women have proven themselves capable of fulfilling any job, including the ones previously thought only suitable for men. It is a blessed common understanding. Indeed, the opening of the western world for women's equality actually happened… or did it?

Here she is, a young, intelligent, ambitious girl, with a career horizon in her mind in the profession she aimed for. Furthermore, she also aims for promotion, which gives her status in society. Her economic situation, however, is an issue sitting in the back of her mind. Female executives are assertive, intelligent and nurtured… and with regard to pregnancy and children, there are two cases: the single woman and the married one.

A single woman thriving in her career; she is over thirty years of age, would like to get married and she is dating. Now, there's a catch. Men are no more self-confident than women. Remember that they deal with their own fears, just as our young lady does. How a person looks is important, but what really counts is assertiveness, brains and business acumen. She sets out on a date, wanting to impress him and he shrinks… or he wants to impress her and take over the conversation. Of course, she assesses him as potential father material, but, most importantly, if he is a career man, it means she will have to stop her career ambitions, at least for a period of time. If he is not a career man, status issues will come to the fore. Finding the right man is not so simple. Thoughts constantly arise… should I put my career on hold? Will he be there for me? I worked hard to achieve my status and I am not willing to risk losing it…

And here's the married lady: she wants a family, but her

marriage is not balanced. The relationship with her husband is not good, the communication and the balance at home are not good, so one of the questions that may emerge is whether or not she should have a child, put her career on hold, and if she does that, will he support her reliably, both practically and financially?

Ruth was thirty-five years old and married for three years. The reason she came to me was that she could not conceive. She had undergone three IVF procedures with no success. In the beginning, I aimed to find the blockage in her mind based on childhood events shaping a pregnancy fear blockage. However, very quickly I realized that her marriage might be the main problem.

Her husband was a career man and very self-centered. If she called him during the day, he would be very short with her, sometimes shouting over the phone that he was busy and demanding to know why she was disturbing him. Ruth was also an executive; however, she was also very maternal. She tended to reduce heated situations, not intensify them, using calming techniques and strategies. The stress of the relationship, which also continued at home, brought them to a shutdown in the sense that she developed a fear and needed a barrier from her husband. Having said that, she also loved him and wanted to stay in the relationship. Ruth had troubling thoughts, not only of how he might treat her during pregnancy, but also if he would treat the child as he treated her. This was the main reason. Of course, all along, the financial issue troubled her - that if she had a child, how she would survive, having suspended her career, if he should ever leave her. Ruth started to fade out...

There is no doubt that, if you have a demanding job and a baby at home, life is not simple. If one has a supportive spouse, the problem will not exist. However, if one has a turbulent marriage, it can sometimes be worse than being by oneself. A career has benefits. You can afford a good and comfortable life. And in the back of almost every person's mind, there are thoughts about what will happen to them in old age if they have no money. This fear drives people to develop anxieties regarding their financial situation. An executive needs to juggle between her need for financial security and having a child - to fulfil her mothering instinct - while recognizing that a child is expensive to raise.

Happiness has nothing to do with money, yet, in our material world, money cannot be dismissed as irrelevant. Hence, we have a conflict: on the one hand, to fulfill oneself, which means position and money; on the other, to stop and have a child. The answer is simple. If you want to be a mother, be one. If you are a talented career person, you will be able to return to the circle of work with no problem, together with a child.

Remember that all the positive reactions you get regarding your looks, ability and intelligence may create subconscious expectations for the need to hear it day after day. Allegedly, if you have a child, you risk giving it all up. As long as you are dependent on uplifting surroundings, you will not extract your real inner power. This is your life. You decide what you want, and as long as you do not hurt anyone, every decision you make should serve only you, regardless of what other people think.

So, what can you do?

There are many variants regarding executives. Are you single or married? Your financial situation and lifestyle may produce blocking fears. Another question is how strongly you want to be a mother. The biological clock is no doubt a major factor when you examine your life timetable.

Think of the following question: if I have a baby, what do I lose and what do I gain? Of course, you should look at your financial situation, the help you have from family and friends, and your options when you can go back to work. Remember, the most important person in the world is you. Having a baby is entirely in your hands. Now try to clarify various factors: husband, work, finding a husband or any other barrier over which your mind poses a question mark.

If you were capable of holding down a job before you were a mother, you will have no problem holding down a job after you've become a mother. If you think what you lose in terms of your career, think what you gain in your life.

A firm you work for could go bankrupt, or you might have to leave... but your baby will never tell you that you are not his mother. It's your decision to be a young (or less young) mother, but remember, there may be a moment when you become a CEO, but even with all that power in your hands, your body will tell you that you're too late.

Back to Ruth. The treatment took a turn for the better when the husband came to me, willing to accept that he had personal issues. I walked him through a therapy process. He was an executive, but low self-esteem caused him to cope based on his position and not his abilities. He was a brave person; he was willing to admit and confront his fears very quickly, and Ruth joined us every third session. He loved her, and gradually, with a lot of courage, he became a supportive husband. At this point, Ruth and her husband could examine all the implications of Ruth stopping working for a period, and they came to an understanding and agreed on their options. The next step was to treat Ruth for her abandonment phobia together with her, now supportive, husband. I gave them exercises. The most difficult was that she would text him or call him, and he would not respond. She was not allowed to call him during the day, not at his parents', nor at his office. At the end of the day, it was up to her husband in what way he arrived home - casual, with flowers, with tickets to the theater or any choice. It went wonderfully well. Excitement came into their life, along with positive energies and laughter; their sex life reached new levels.

It was not long before Ruth conceived naturally. She had a fantastic support from her exhilarated husband, and six months after the birth she went back to work.

Now, Ruth sees the world from a different perspective: as a mother. She no longer aims for the highest job. Rather, she wants to bring more children into the world and remain in the working circle, but at a level that will allow her to enjoy her role as a mother and wife.

Babyphobia

OVER THIRTY AND STILL SINGLE

Shiran was a thirty-four-year-old computer programmer. She had a good job along with a good income, her own apartment and she was healthy.

Well, what went wrong? No man on the scene...

On the one hand, Shiran was an average looking girl, and on the other, a smart and balanced person. Her life was a bit on the quiet side - no clubbing, nothing extreme, no one night stands. She was just looking for the right guy with whom to create a harmonious relationship and get married. She had enjoyed a few relationships during her life, however, none of them progressed to living together and getting married.

Natasha was thirty-five and worked in an administrative job. Financially, she was okay. Natasha was a very attractive woman, she liked flirting, the good life, dancing, and traveling... but Natasha was drifting between a few men. She needed two main things: courting and compliments - and a magnificently built man. All of her relationships started with sparks and lightning; however, none of the men ever took any action to establish their relationship.

There are approximately fifty million unmarried women over the age of eighteen in the United States. Of those, more than six million are between the ages of thirty-five and forty.

No, I do not discuss how to get married; I lay out your conflicts when your mind and body are telling you that they want a baby. There is no doubt that your biological clock is ticking, and getting pregnant at the age of forty is not as easy as it is at twenty-five. Your mind is in turmoil. You want a spouse - one who suits you both as a woman and as a supportive father. Finding the correct man is not simple. There are many issues when two people meet, and finding a spouse with whom you want to share your life is also a question of luck. On the other hand, you do not want to stop looking until you find Mr. Right.

So, what can you do?

In order to level your thoughts and understand your choices in life, you first need to understand your values in life. What are the important things in your life? You need to grade them and understand what the most important things are for you now, and comprehend the less important things in your current life.

Often, we connect to a person because we have a spark, usually physical; we all know the story - three months of ecstasy, falling in love involving mainly a physical connection… but then, when we need to build our love life, the dialogue, to contain the other and balance the relationship, it falls apart.

There are ways to go about this: the better way, the way that will hurt you less, the way that can nurture a healthy relationship. When you meet a guy, you first need to see if his physique and looks please you, but be warned - if he repulses you, do not proceed. However, even if he is not your Dream Come True - only okay - do not reject him out of hand. So you sit together to have coffee, to find out who this person is, his history, what he likes in terms of traveling, spare time, friends, sports, etc. If you like only five stars hotels, but he likes only sleeping with nature, you already have a big problem, no matter how he looks. If you like to eat out a lot or go out every night, while he likes to be at home more, think again. There are many such things that define people. You don't need to conduct an interview, but you do need to see if the person facing you answers questions freely, faces your questions, and doesn't change the subject. Body language and eye contact are important factors. The principle is, after the stage of liking the look, you need to shut down your emotions and use your cognitive area to understand if the person sitting in front of you has any potential from the point of view of life values. If the first date goes okay, and you are happy to see him for a second date, it is going well. Again, you dig deeper into this person (not like a police interrogation, but in free conversation) and can find out a lot about the person in front of you. Women have intuition, so use it.

By this time, you may feel comfortable with this person, so now you can allow a small feeling to grow toward him.

It should take some time... text messages and phone conversations that establish not only a trust toward this person, but also feelings. Do things together, including sex, though preferably not before the fifth date. If, after having sex, he continues his courtship and his behavior is still courteous and warm, then now you are in a healthy relationship with a person who wants the same life as you, including children and a mutual life.

Finding such a person is not simple. You need to be strong, not just be driven by lust without a cognitive understanding of why you are there. No doubt, luck plays a role when looking for a spouse.

What should you do if the knight is not to be found? If the biological clock is ticking? Be brave. Set a target date, by which time, if you have not found a life partner, then get pregnant and have a child. The regret and sorrow if you miss the opportunity will make you an old, bitter fifty-year-old woman. Treasure the happiness you can give yourself, and if, along the way, the right person joins you, he is welcome. After all, you are a sweet person with a sweet baby.

Back to Shiran and Natasha.

Shiran was very cooperative during the therapy process; she really faced it with courage, confronted her fears and avoided dark thoughts. She became almost indifferent to dating. Her will to have a baby was so strong that she deserved a miracle; a suitable man should have appeared on the scene, but did not. At a certain point, she decided to be a single mother. She got pregnant using a sperm bank, and she now has a year-old baby. Nothing can be compared to the happiness she experienced and the understanding that she made the right choice for herself. Now she is dating, but from a different angle. Now she has an anchor waiting for her at home. If the date is disappointing, at least she will never return home to empty rooms.

Natasha started slowly, but with a lot of courage, progressed through the therapy. Her task was to do the opposite in real life, like looking in a mirror. Systematically, she understood what she had done wrong in previous relationships, but after a while, she found another escape, submitting to her lust and unrealistic dreams. Natasha also had mild epilepsy. When she was in an exciting and pleasing situation, she did not suffer any fits, but the moment her man started to avoid her or made excuses not to see her, she had multiple attacks due to stress. During the therapy, she slowly ceased to have attacks, and became more relaxed, but once she stopped, the fits returned, a direct result of the stress she put herself under, despite her knowledge of things she knew she should do, as opposed to the wrong things she actually did. Natasha is still single, frustrated and unable to create clear decisions regarding her life. She is still drifting.

These days, thirty may be the new twenty, but a woman's reproductive system remains as ever it was. The social stress on a single woman intensifies as she grows older. When she reaches the stage where her friends are pregnant or already have babies, stress starts to control her life, asking "what if" questions. This process creates fears of negative self-esteem and a sense of urgency, like the white rabbit in *Alice in Wonderland*. If a woman has family members with babies, the stress will intensify every time she sees them, hugs them, and smells them, wishing this baby was hers.

There are hundreds of books and guides telling you how to find a life partner - your knight on a white horse.

As I mentioned above, finding a spouse depends primarily on you - understanding who you are, what you want from life, how you see potential life partners, what essential qualities they must have, and what you may agree to compromise on. Finally, it depends on your courage to implement decisions in your life.

Having a baby by yourself does not in any way suggest failure. On the contrary, it tells the world that you are a brave woman, a woman who does not want to compromise on her fears, a woman who understands that her biological clock has a baby-expiration date, and a woman who wants to be a mother. For you, the rest of the world is irrelevant to your happiness, which you created by yourself, for yourself.

Babyphobia

SPERM BANK ISSUES

When Rachel set an appointment with me, I could hear her tears over the phone. She told me that she had already been in therapy for two years, but no change had happened in her life. She was thirty-five. When I opened the door, I saw a smiling pretty face. She was somewhat rotund.

Rachel was a very bright woman who had a very clear vision of the world surrounding her, along with the great frustration of not finding a man to marry.

There is a point in her life when a woman decides to have a baby, regardless of whether or not she has a partner, or even if her partner has no fertile sperm. This stage is already the end of a long journey. However, what is happening in her life prior to this might be the most significant decision she has ever taken in her life.

She has probably been through a few years during which she dated, had partners, and nurtured dreams, but none of them materialized. In terms of fertility, perhaps she is no longer young and the window for being pregnant is narrowing. More than that. She has thoughts of how young a mother she will be. If she conceives when she is, say, forty-two, she will not be a young mother. She contemplates, since she is by herself - at least for now - thoughts of what will come of her baby if something happened to her. How will she function as a sixty-year-old mother to a twenty-year-old? The thoughts go back and forth like a game of ping-pong, delaying her decision.

The questions we raise about what will happen in the future are mostly very irrelevant. We cannot guess the future and it is very dangerous to speculate about things over which we have no control. "What if?" questions are relevant only to things we have a firm option about: if I call a friend I can say, "If you come over, I'll make you a nice cup of coffee." So, if he comes over, I'll make coffee, and if not, then I won't. When we program software, we use the statement "if." That is how computers work, although a computer's knowledge is preset and not open to speculation. When we look at life, and speculate about the future, we take risks. For example: I'm thirty-eight years of age... I want a baby... I'm considering going to the sperm bank to conceive... but *what if* a month after I conceive, I meet the man of my dreams, and because I'm pregnant he rejects me... what will happen?

It is all about things no one ever promised us - but yet, we are afraid to lose them.

Another "if": what if I go to the sperm bank, and I conceive, but the sperm I get is that of an unintelligent person, or he had a genetic problem to hide?

Our minds can generate endless scenarios if we have life blocking fears. Those fears can go in various directions - for instance, self-pity, declaring that you are a failure, because you did not find a husband and resorted to the sperm bank like a loser. You need to agree with yourself about one thing: I have the right to create something good for myself and I am the most important person in the world.

So, what can you do?

The first thing to understand is that you have a biological clock. You need to avoid being stressed. Stress makes you uneasy, forcing you to take the wrong decision. When you think calmly, time passes slowly. When you are relaxed, you are able to understand your situation, the questions you have, and the options before you.

If you do not find a life partner, yet you do not want to give up your life values, then you may come to the point at which you tell yourself this: a husband would be nice, but what I really want is a baby and it is in my power and under my control to do that. It often happens that single mothers find a partner a short time after having a baby. It is not a promise; however, there is a reason for it. Many self-anxieties regarding self-values, fear of failure, fear of abandonment, and others, will be gone when you have a baby. At this point in your life, you have an anchor at home. No matter what happens when you go on a date, you always have your anchor at home; thus, your anxieties do not lead you. It is up to you to decide when you want to stop waiting for the shining knight on the white horse. If you can afford to, have some of your eggs frozen and go for an IVF process whenever you decide is the right time. It has been proven that the quality of a woman's eggs will decrease as she ages. Think of a moment of your life as one important evening, an important occasion. You prepare yourself in every respect. You sleep well, get your hair done, find a special dress and shoes, and apply your makeup with great care. Now, take a step backwards and look at your life. See the options, prepare the aspects of life you are responsible for, evaluate those options, and set a date at which you will activate your chosen options.

Back to Rachel. Her body image created a defense area when she was intimate with a man. Of course, this obstacle also reflected on her behavior while dating. During our therapy process, Rachel started to accept herself. No, she did not delude herself that she had the perfect body, but she was less and less troubled by her body. She even started to like some parts and accepted her other parts as something she was born with, and as part of her. Now, when she dated, her cognitive area was working stronger, and she was better able to analyze if her date was the right person for her.

In our world today, dating is far from simple. On the one hand, one can find anything over the Internet. However, finding a true person - the right one - is not so simple. We go back to the decision of how long to wait, and contemplate life with kids and no husband. Rachel decided that freezing her eggs may encourage procrastination and she might postpone the decision until a point at which it might be too late. Therefore, she set a timetable for her life, and was firm to lead herself according to this timetable with a lot of courage.

After evaluating all variables, the one she had no control over, and the ones she did have control over, Rachel decided to go to a sperm bank. She went through the procedure, and was successful. Her pregnancy was normal and she gave birth to a healthy baby girl. Well, the little girl has blue eyes and Rachel's are brown, so, okay, that's a chance you have to take when you go to the sperm bank.

THE "L" WORD

Tanya was thirty-two and studying for her M.A. in Paramedicine. She told me that the reason she came to me was that she had problems with her relationship with her girlfriend. They shared an apartment. They did not share the same room; however, they often slept together. The relationship was very tense. Her partner was often insulted by things Tanya could not understand, and often made controlling remarks about Tanya's dress, especially when they went out to have a drink at a gay/lesbian club. There was love and good sex, but also envy and control that made Tanya frustrated and induced depression and an inability to understand what to do.

Being homosexual or lesbian is not necessarily set from birth. Why? Since the reasons for a woman becoming lesbian are many, and those reasons have an effect when two women decide to live together and have a baby.

Many heterosexual women are curious about experiencing sex with a woman and often contemplate it at different stages in their lives. Many women on the rebound after experiencing a ruined relationship with a man will try a sexual relationship with a woman; some of them will stay with a woman for the rest of their life. In addition, I am not forgetting the girls who know almost from the beginning that they are attracted to other women, and who have no doubts about their sexuality. The more important issue is that in most countries today, they do not have to hide, and in some countries they can get married, the law regarding lesbian marriages being the same as those between men and women.

Women are more emotional. This is a biological fact. The brain structure of a woman's brain hemispheres is different from that of a man, which are connected by countable connections, but with women they are almost one unit. It is no exaggeration to say that every word a woman says is combined with emotion; even a simple "Good morning" comes from different areas of the brain from men's. One other important factor is the hormones.

When a man develops, his main hormone is testosterone, and the journey of a boy to a man is reflected in his bodily development. When a boy becomes an adult, he is the same, but bigger. A girl has a very different journey. At a certain stage, her body starts to transform. One day, without warning, she will get her first period, and from then on, she is fertile. Hormonal activity in women causes moodiness. Therefore, women may have problems understanding the outcome of hormonal activity.

The mind cannot monitor every biological and emotional activity and create a cognitive report. There are claims that women are smarter than men. Perhaps they are, but there is no doubt that women are much more complicated machines than men, both physically and emotionally. When two women start a relationship, it is like any other relationship with the chemistry, the electricity in the air, the conversation and all the tools needed for a relationship. Now, a hidden trap awaits. They can be very understanding and have great empathy for one another, but sometimes this understanding can be an obstacle if the hormonal activity between them is very different. The mental build of a woman makes her more sensitive, thus, the results of bad or good outcomes are intensified. During arguments, stress levels can reach the sky. Jealousy is also intensified in a lesbian relationship. The words "You don't understand me!" take on a very different meaning inside a lesbian relationship than when they are thrown at a man. Like in every relationship, there is usually one dominant partner, and one who is more loving. It is not necessarily the same person.

After all the universal difficulties of finding a life partner, they are in a good, balanced lesbian relationship. They share an apartment and conduct a normal life together. Now they are in love, and both of them want to take the relationship to the next step. In some cases, only one of them may want a baby, while the other does not. In some cases both of them might like to have a baby.

However, when they are both girls, an unexpected pregnancy cannot happen. If they want a baby, they need to look outside their relationship. Technically, there are two options: a male volunteer, or a sperm bank.

Now they take it to the next level.

Like any couple, there is no guarantee that their relationship will last forever. Now, I refer them to the chapter *Over Thirty and Still Single*. If they want a baby, they should not let any fears over abandonment or finance stop them. They should go and get a donor and have a baby. Like any couple, if they live together long enough, married or not, they are recognized as common-law spouses.

If they think about what is stopping them from having a baby, they will find the same reason as in every turbulent relationship. If their relationship is good, they shouldn't hesitate to have a baby, but, what if the process fails, time after time, when they are healthy and do not understand why?

The mental barriers stopping a woman from getting pregnant are many, and even more so in a lesbian relationship because most lesbian couples are not married, do not have mutual assets and they are both in the same situation. Their questions and anxieties increase when the issue of a baby arises.

So, what can you do?

This is the time to examine your fears sitting in the back of your mind... all the "what if" questions. Write them down in two columns: the things that are under your control and the things that are not. Now, erase all things that are not under your control and examine the list. You will find that the remaining items in your list are the ones that will create happiness and fulfillment in your life. Do not forget, the fact that you are in a lesbian relationship does not change the fact that you might want to fulfill your life as a mother. All other elements such as envy, control, jealousy and others are artificial and they should not stop you.

What if you want to stay with your female partner, but you want to conceive from a male friend? The "what if" questions are endless. Think of any male/female relationship; they get married. Having a baby is almost expected from them, so no one will be surprised if, two months after marriage, the woman is pregnant. On the contrary, everyone will congratulate her. Reflect it back on you. If you want to be a mother, erase all the "what if" questions concerning the fact that you have a female partner, and just go ahead and do it. Being a mother has nothing to do with what your preferences are, but being a mother is your natural born right.

When you want to decide on something that big in your life, it is very important to contemplate what happens the day after you deliver your baby. If you conceived from a man, he may want to be involved in the child's life, and want to know how he will be included, and whether he can come and see the baby, or take the baby for the day. All of that must be discussed and agreed upon; more important is your spouse's agreement. Do not forget that whoever delivers the baby, their partner will feel that you are a family, sharing tasks including those to do with the baby. The male donor man could pose a threat to this cozy unit.

Even if you agree to go through an IVF process with an unknown donor, the baby is still yours. If your partner is fertile and plans to have a baby of her own in the future, you must establish this understanding with her after you bring the baby home.

What happened to Tanya? During the therapy, she realized that her current relationship was created from her own fears. She understood that her current spouse was actually stopping her from life fulfillment in every respect. Tanya took a brave decision; she separated from her partner and moved to her own place. The mourning stage of the separation did not stop her from restarting her life. She managed to complete her M.A. After she regained her self-confidence, she started dating again, this time equipped with tools enabling her to make fewer mistakes. She met a girl of her own age. They started to date; Tanya had a good job by now in her field. She was relaxed; anger and frustration did not appear in her life any more. After about six months, they decided to share the same roof. They discussed the "what if we separate" question. Tanya told me that they wanted to eliminate any potential separation issue. They decided to get the best from all worlds. The most amazing thing happened... *both* went through an IVF process, *both* got pregnant, and they gave birth one week apart... and as an added benefit, both their families could help much more because they now had two families. This was an amazing result for two brave women.

The cry of a newborn baby is the most wonderful sound a human being ever produced.

Babyphobia

CHILDHOOD ABUSE

Child abuse is categorized into three types: physical, mental and sexual.

These types of abuse have subcategories, but for the purpose of our subject matter, the main categories will be sufficient. There are, of course, one-time traumas that can be projected at a later age that affect pregnancy, however, those traumas can emerge from endless events, hence, they cannot be discussed here. In any case, most life blockages occur during known events as I stated above. The process is: abuse leading to trauma and then to PTSD. In most cases, the effect of the trauma will be reflected in different guises from the actual events that happened in early age.

PHYSICAL ABUSE

The impact of physical abuse in childhood on adults is less severe than that of mental or sexual abuse. A woman who suffered physical abuse in childhood can develop phobias or anxieties in adulthood. Physical traumas can affect pregnancy without any connection to abuse. A woman traumatized by needles or doctors as a child can develop a fear of what will happen to her during labor, and this could be enough to prevent her from becoming pregnant.

The effects of physical abuse vary in relation to a woman's sexuality and pregnancy. A woman can submit herself to BDSM relationships due to physical abuse. Alternatively, she may completely avoid physical contact as an adult.

A woman who has experienced physical abuse as a child needs to understand that body image, self-esteem, fear of authority and more can create a phobia about pregnancy. It is not the pregnancy itself; it is the child, and what will happen to him. The thoughts of the past block the body from its future.

MENTAL ABUSE

Modern research suggests that the impact of mental abuse is as great as that of sexual abuse, though the effects in adulthood are not the same. Mental abuse mostly creates low self-evaluation - a sense of being unworthy. This may reflect as fear of authority, but mainly as fear of failure. When a woman grows up concerned about what the people around her think of her, she also expects positive reactions to what she does, or what she wears. Her mind is mainly concerned with how she looks to the people she comes into contact with; she may be very helpful to friends, even if she has to put herself out, as long as she hears how wonderful a person and friend she is. Then, the same trauma can expand to: "I do not deserve..." She might find it difficult to give to herself. When we discuss pregnancy, her mind might say, "I deserve..." but immediately after, it asks her what will happen if she fails? How people will react?" She needs to learn how to agree to fail. She needs to remember that mental traumas are not as strong as real DNA. In severe cases, I have encountered young women whose periods stopped due to extreme low self-esteem, which led to eating disorders causing physical outcomes that prevented them from conceiving.

SEXUAL ABUSE

The following is a quote from a research study I conducted regarding child abuse and the potential for a balanced life for an abused child. The method I developed, Rebound Psychotherapy, has proved to succeed in "balancing" woman abused in childhood, including solving pregnancy issues and achieving a balanced family life.

"Research has established that adverse early life experiences, particularly sexual abuse, may cause major depression disorders including PTSD. As a result, people who were sexually abused in childhood are exposed to chronic life stress that can lead to depression, suicidal tendencies, loss of libido and promiscuity. We also learned that environmental conditions such as mother/father relationships, brother/sister relationships, the socioeconomic situation and the cultural/societal environment are significant factors in the after results of the abuse."

Rose was twenty-four when I met her; she had been married for two years.

During the therapy process, I found that Rose suffered from a certain degree of paranoia, her periods were not regular, she had anxiety about abandonment and she had very low self-esteem.

Rose was an only child; during the day, her father worked, but the mother was the homemaker. Rose's mother often went out of the house for a variety of reasons - shopping, meeting with friends and more - and during that time, her brother looked after Rose. This uncle was nineteen years old. We started to go back to her childhood, but Rose's memories went back only to the age of seven.

The uncle was not aggressive. He lured Rose slowly by being tender, warm and understanding, and he gave her small gifts and slowly managed to have physical contact with her. To begin with, it involved some touching, including her vagina. The peak of the abuse was an oral act by Rose on her uncle, and having her intimate parts touched, including finger penetration.

During the therapy, I uncovered two major issues that significantly affected Rose's life. The first was that her mother did not allow her to cry. Under no circumstances, even if she was sad, hurt or insulted, was she allowed to cry. This fact led Rose into an emotional deprivation that made her uncle's task much easier. Rose needed love and attention and he identified that and gave her what she missed. The other issue was that Rose's mother denied her brother's actions. All through Rose's life, up to the present day, whenever she tried to confront her mother regarding her uncle's actions, her mother dismissed it, saying that it was not possible and that it was a figment of her imagination.

Indeed, a percentage of the girls who suffered from sexual abuse as children grow up to be balanced women who can create a balanced life and enjoy a family.

However, the majority of sexually abused girls walk a very bumpy road. All of us, as children, experience trauma during our development. A trauma can be a one-off event such as one seeing one's dog run down by a car, or a trauma suffered while trying out new things as a toddler, which could have happened regularly. If you come home from school with only a moderate exam result, and your mother or father repeatedly tells you that you could do better, this creates a trauma, which will lead to fear of failure and low self-esteem. The epigenetic cells in our brains accumulate emotional barriers, blocking some of our DNA (usually the emotional part, but not only; autoimmunity can be affected). For most people, the mental barriers or fears created by the epigenetic cells will not block them from having a fairly balanced life. Additionally, some of our fears can disappear due to life experience. People under the age of eighteen who go to see therapists usually manage to improve their lives more easily than adults, since the brain is still developing.

Sexual abuse is no doubt amongst the most severe abuses a child can experience. The results of sexual abuse, as I mentioned above, can be suicidal tendencies, constant depression, avoidance of sex and physical touch, or promiscuity.

Through guilt and shame, many sexually abused women just suppress the events, live in denial and suffer from fear and life-blocking thoughts without understanding why. Most sexually abused women feel guilt and shame about what happened. Even adult women who are victims of rape feel guilty about the event.

There is a reason why legislation defines the term "under age." The reason is that "under aged" people are not fully responsible for their actions. Why? Two reasons: firstly, the brain is not yet fully functional; and secondly, they do not have enough information to analyze the events. Under age, the brain is still in the learning process. However, as a grown-up, judgement may come from the adult's cognitive area and criticize the child for what happened in the past. This is one of the reasons for suppressing the past, since the adult knows that what happened was wrong, and today she would not agree to such an act; hence comes the inner struggle between the epigenetic area in the back of our minds and our adult cognitive area. The result is that, since the cognitive area is in denial, the adult will avoid dealing with the pain and will flee to other places such as depression and other issues I mentioned above. Significantly, a biological blockage will stop her body from conceiving.

So, what can you do?

The first thing: understand that what happened to you as a child was not your fault. You have nothing to be ashamed of. Understand that the person who did that to you is/was mentally sick. You did not choose to be there, and you were a hostage.

Agree that you suffer from a disturbance that escorts you constantly on a daily basis. Try to remember your childhood events and the abuse you suffered. This is very important. If you are reading this and you are under eighteen, do this with the aid of a therapist - not by yourself.

You were under age. Even if you were exploited because you missed affection, and your abuser gave you a hug, it is *still* not your fault. If your abuser intimidates you – I repeat: he took advantage of a child without the tools to fully understand the events.

Even prison inmates go through rehabilitation; they pay their debt to society and they are then allowed to return to society rehabilitated, so a different person goes back out into the world. You are now a grown-up, you are no longer a frightened kid; you need to understand that should your abuser try to do today what he did in the past, you would not let him. In some cases, the abuser is the father, and in those cases, sometimes the mother knew but did nothing. It is up to you if you choose to hate or to forgive, and it is up to you to materialize as a strong, independent person, who makes her own choices today.

Your life today is not a reflection of the past, but a creation of your present day, adult decisions.

It's time to get a therapist to help and identify for you in what way the abuse reflects on your life today - if it is low self-esteem, fear of authority, body image or anything else. You will have to start a dialog with your fears. The next step is to move yourself to a different space from the one you are in now. In this a different space, where you will need to face things blocked in the past by your fears. Remember the things you are afraid of, and write them down. Now choose the least frightening one, the one that looks the easiest, and face it. First, it will take a while to achieve, and you will try and avoid it, but once you succeed in making the first step, you are on the right track.

Balancing yourself may take a long time. Your ultimate aim is to be a mother. Try yourself, or with help, to identify and differentiate what is stopping you from conceiving, and what is irrelevant. After you become a mother, some of your other fears may disappear by themselves. It is not mandatory for anyone to eliminate all the fears in life. The main thing is that we should treat the fears stopping us from fulfilling important goals we set ourselves in life.

Back to Rose. I asked her to bring her husband along. After I met him, I realized that Rose had received a gift.

He was tender, understanding, with no aggression or frustration at all, just the will to help as he could. One of Rose's problems was freezing during sex. She did not experience orgasms, but she did pamper her husband, however. She had no notion regarding the words "I deserve…" I started to work with Rose, first on her self-esteem in the outside world, in the street, with her friend, at work. I also minimized her conversations with her mother as to what was happening in her life. Her mother was a very dominant controlling person, and was used to questioning Rose about her life, telling her what to do and judging her. She never did accept Rose's story of abuse.

After about four months, Rose started to stabilize and became more vital; she smiled more and became more independent. Now, the point arrived at which I started talking with her about her body, about sex and her sexual relationship with her husband. Slowly, with her husband's help, Rose learned to release control during sex, to lie on her back and let her husband pamper her. Two months later, Rose's periods returned to normal, and after her third regular period, Rose conceived and she gave birth naturally.

Rose is a very brave woman who accepted having a dialog with the little Rose hiding in the back of her mind, and accepted herself, together with her strong, adult being.

We cannot erase memories. We can try to suppress memories; however, doing so will cause us constant stress. We should remember not only the good things, but also the bad things. We need to understand what happened to us in the past, and create tools based on our past.

Being brave is admitting a failure; being happy is to build a world based on who you really are.

Babyphobia

EPILOGUE: YOUR NEXT STEP

Nothing is impossible and everything is possible… and don't let anyone tell you different.

Just by reading this book, you may consider yourself a brave woman. You have read about reasons, but also about fears. Perhaps you recognized yourself in one of the chapters.

Do not hesitate. You can do it. Try to exercise some of what I suggested. Understand that whatever is blocking your pregnancy was created in your mind long ago, when you were only a child. As a child, you did not have the mental ability, nor the tools to understand that certain events in your childhood would one day create a mental block to conception.

Now, you are a grown-up person. Think of the things you have achieved in your life. Refresh your mind of the events in which you were strong, assertive, funny, brave, a good friend, enjoyed pleasure, got the job you wanted, and bought that car you wanted. Even the smallest things matter… a witty reply you gave, a nice idea for yourself, anything that points to yourself as a leader and not as a follower. Write them down. Now, even if you feel low, you will realize that you have no reason to be. Be proud of yourself, and do not let any opinion change this. Only you can decide who you are. Your life is like driving. Your body is the vehicle you were given, now it's up to you how you drive it.

Life is a collection of events. Space is a collection of events, yet, in this turbulent universe, new stars are born. No matter how your space looks, it's up to you to create a new star: a child of your own.

Babyphobia

ABOUT THE AUTHOR

I was born on 3 December 1954. I was small, had spastic bronchial asthma, and was shy and insecure. When I went to high school, something changed... I got pimples. I also practiced Judo and joined a swimming team. When I was eighteen, I went into the military, which is compulsory in my country. They told me that I was going to be a pilot. I looked for the hidden camera (recording this joke being played on me) but there was no camera. Two years later, I became an air force pilot. As an insecure person blossoming into a very self-confident pilot, I underwent a magnificent journey. In this journey, I was torn between my two selves.

At the age of twenty-seven, two significant events took place in my life: I got lost in Nepal, during an August trek in the Himalayas at 12,000 ft., but caught between life and death, I managed to return; the other was crossing the Nullarbor Desert in Australia, by myself, on a motorcycle.

When I returned, I began my university studies. During the next twelve years, I worked for commercial companies in a variety of jobs, including as a business developer, a contract manager, a CEO and a director.

I was married and divorced. I have two daughters – Adi, twenty-four, and Shani, twenty years old.

When I was forty years old and already divorced, all my life events, emotions, thoughts, and the world, just smashed into my being. I realized that I was living my life wrongly, and I was devastated. I agreed to admit to myself all my mistakes. I agreed to realize and understand who I am, for real. I completely transformed my life from a material lifestyle to one where I sought contentment for myself. Only then did I decide what to take from life, and why.

I knew then that I understand and see into people, but

all my life I advised people from a place of insecurity. I needed to hear from them how smart I was.

I learned to separate the fear from my real ability. I went on to study human behavior, methods of treatment, and finally I earned my Ph.D. The title of my work was: *Child Sexual Abuse and the Ability to Have a Balanced Adult Life*.

For the last twelve years, I have worked as a psychotherapist in my own clinic. I treat healthy women who cannot conceive, as well as anxieties of all types including anxiety stress, fear of flying, agoraphobia and many others. My treatments also include women's sexuality, therapy for couples and for teenagers from fourteen on.

My next step is to conduct a research into OCD, in which I want to prove that treatment can reduce a person's compulsive obsessions. I intend to exercise the treatment system I developed and established, called Rebound Psychotherapy.

Thank you for sharing your time with me.

Tzachi Topelberg Ph.D.

Mail: drtopelberg@gmail.com

Skype: drtopelberg